Rub a Dub Dub
Clean and Scrub

Read & Reminisce

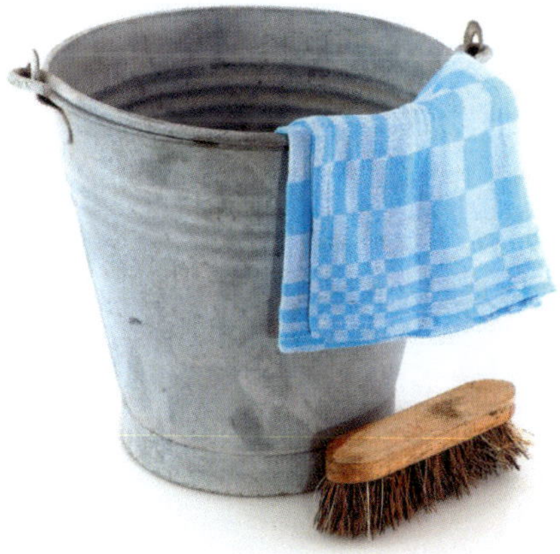

Enjoy these tales of cleaning in the 'good old days'. Maybe you have other stories to share?

Back in the day...

Back in the day, a spotless home was a big source of pride. Kids often got into trouble for tracking in dirt.

Studies show that women spent much more time on home duties than they do now. Yet we had less ‘stuff’ and most houses only had only one bathroom.

Appliances were more basic. There were jobs like defrosting the fridge or sweeping out the grate that now seem a world away... for most of us!

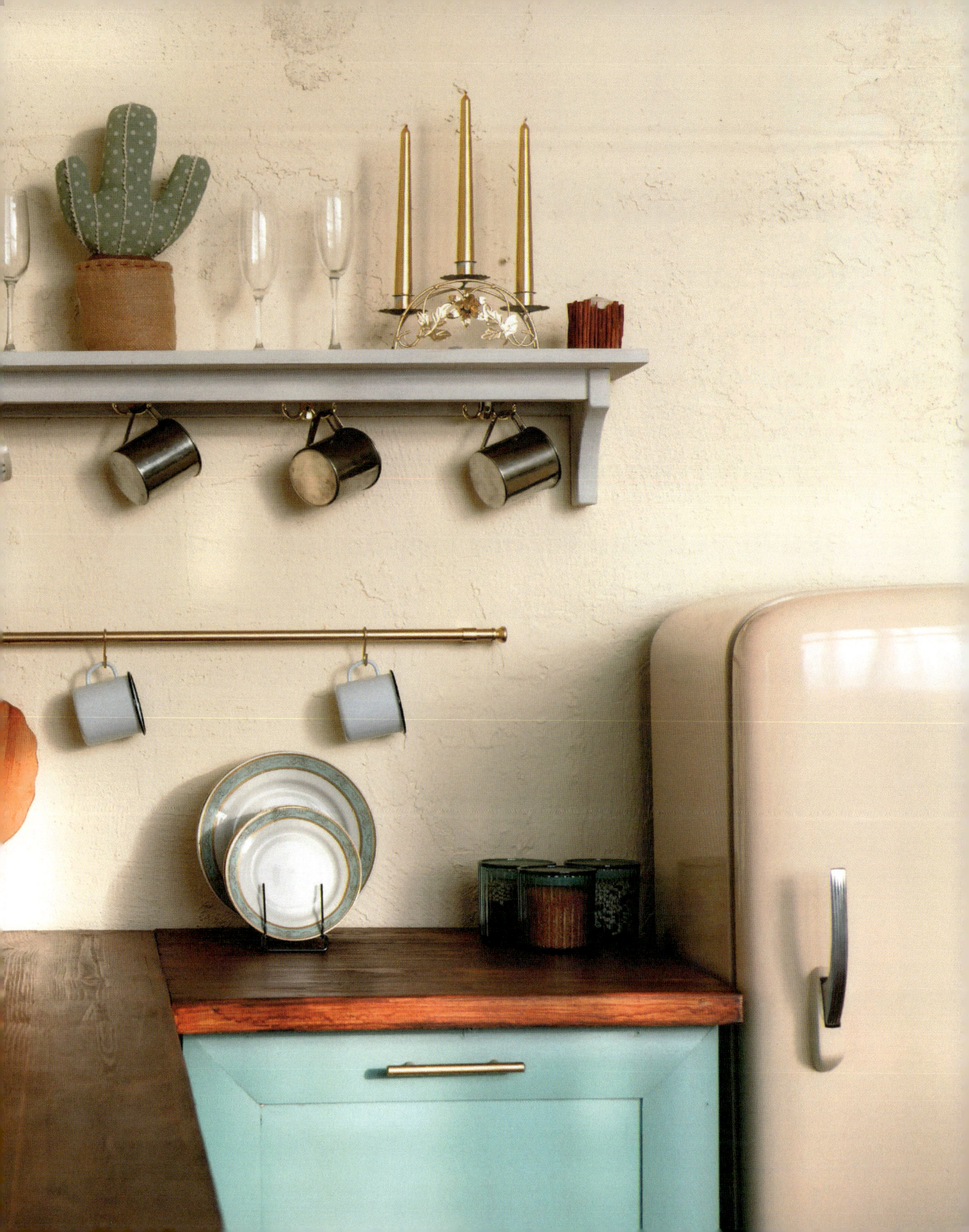

Floors

Who remembers mopping and waxing the floors? Lino or wood, they all got that weekly attention!

For our carpets and rugs, we had a heavy vacuum cleaner or a little carpet sweeper to pick up crumbs. Mats would be hung on the washing line and beaten to get out all the grit.

As with everything, elbow grease was the key ingredient! No need to go to the gym with all that housework!

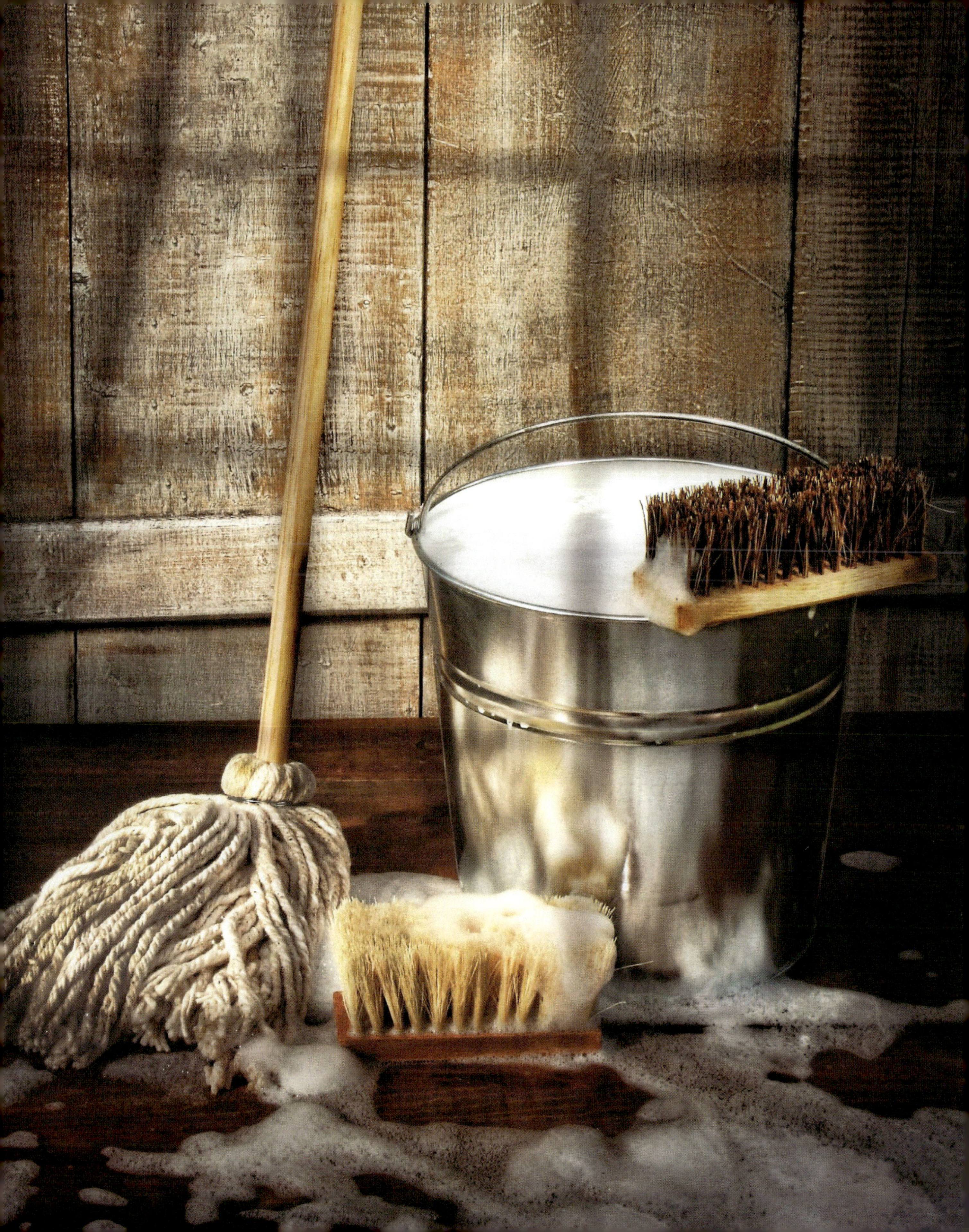

Dust and polish

You dusted with a wet and a dry duster, or with a feather duster. Venetian blinds were a real challenge to keep clean.

There were no microfibre cloths back then, or paper towels, but there was a plentiful supply of rags, made from old clothing.

The wood polish had a lovely pungent smell. Copper pans and ornaments needed regular polishing, and so did any silverware. More of that elbow grease was needed!

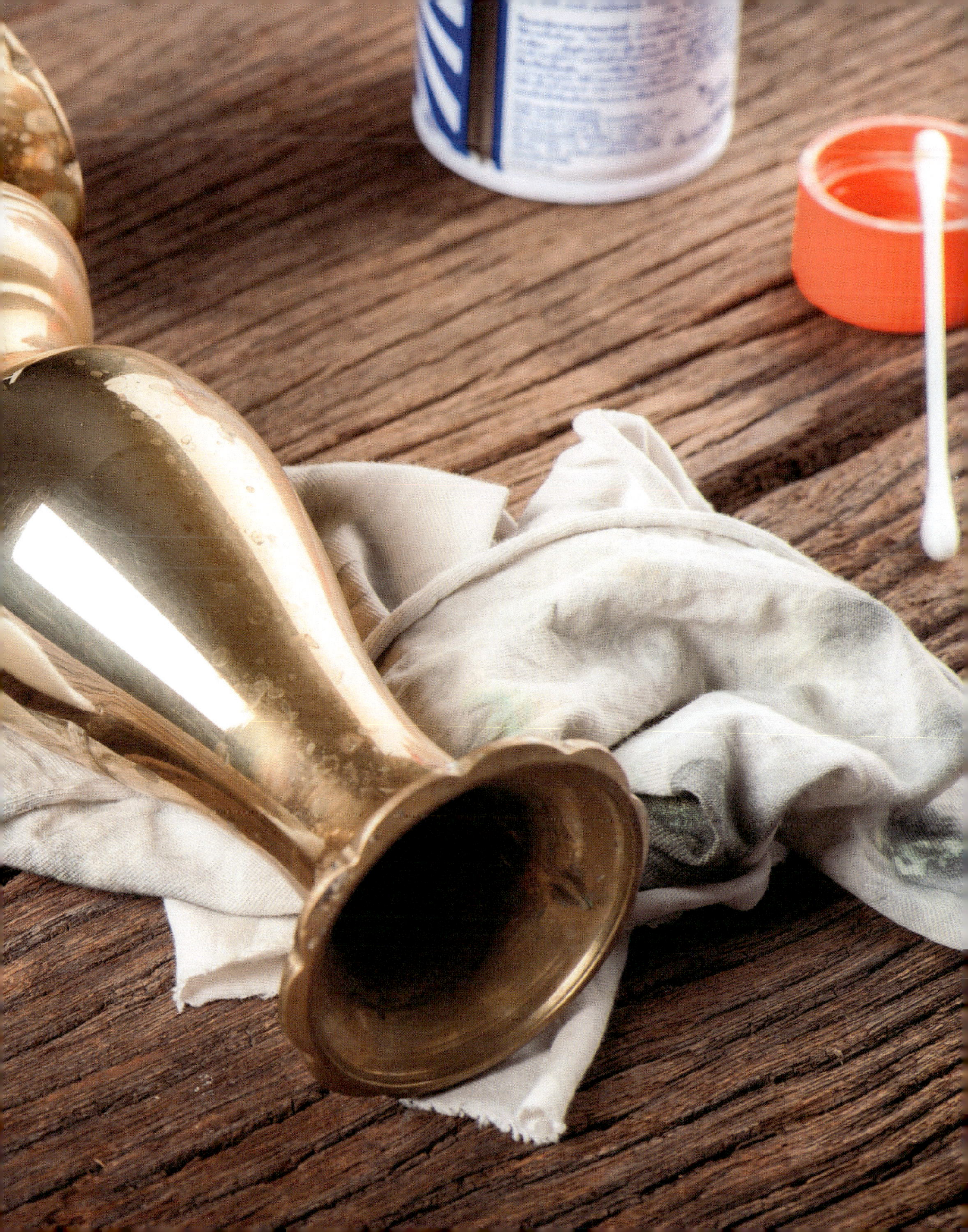

Sparkling clean!

Cupboards back then were full of bleach and ammonia, borax, caustic soda, methylated spirits and washing soda.

That sounds like a lot of chemicals, but plenty of people relied on 'soda bicarb' (baking soda) and vinegar.

You could also say we were 'eco', because we didn't wash every item after only one wear. We simply sponged heavy items, and hung them outside to air.

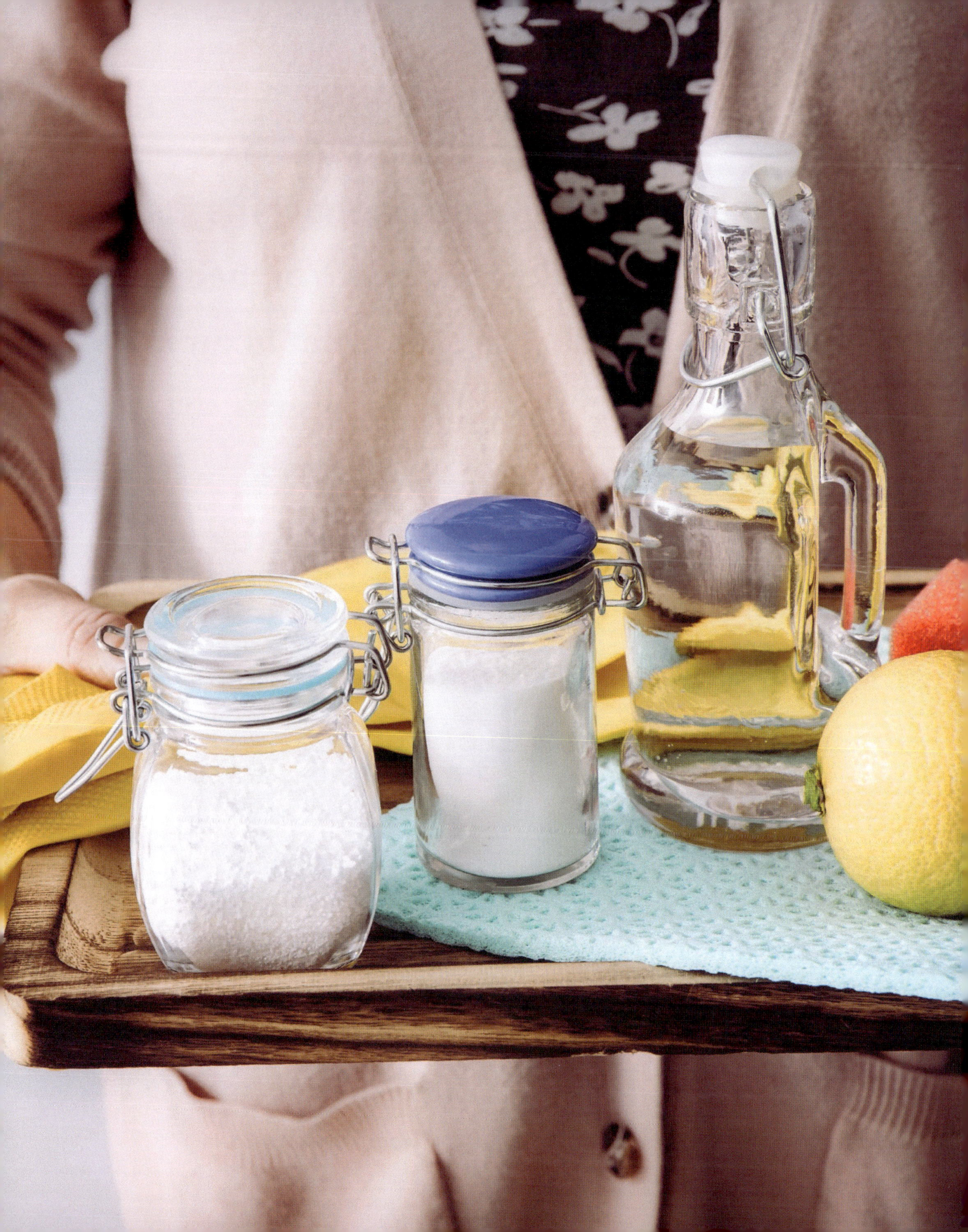

Washing day

Some of us had a washing machine with a wringer, a bit like this one. You had to fill it with a hose, but still, what luxury. No more boiling clothes in a copper!

Others remember the old ‘dolly’ tub and cutting soap from a bar. In our house we used soap flakes from a box, plus a blue bag rinse at the end of the wash.

Some people dipped all their washing in liquid starch, but that eventually went out of style. Still, washing day was a lot of work.

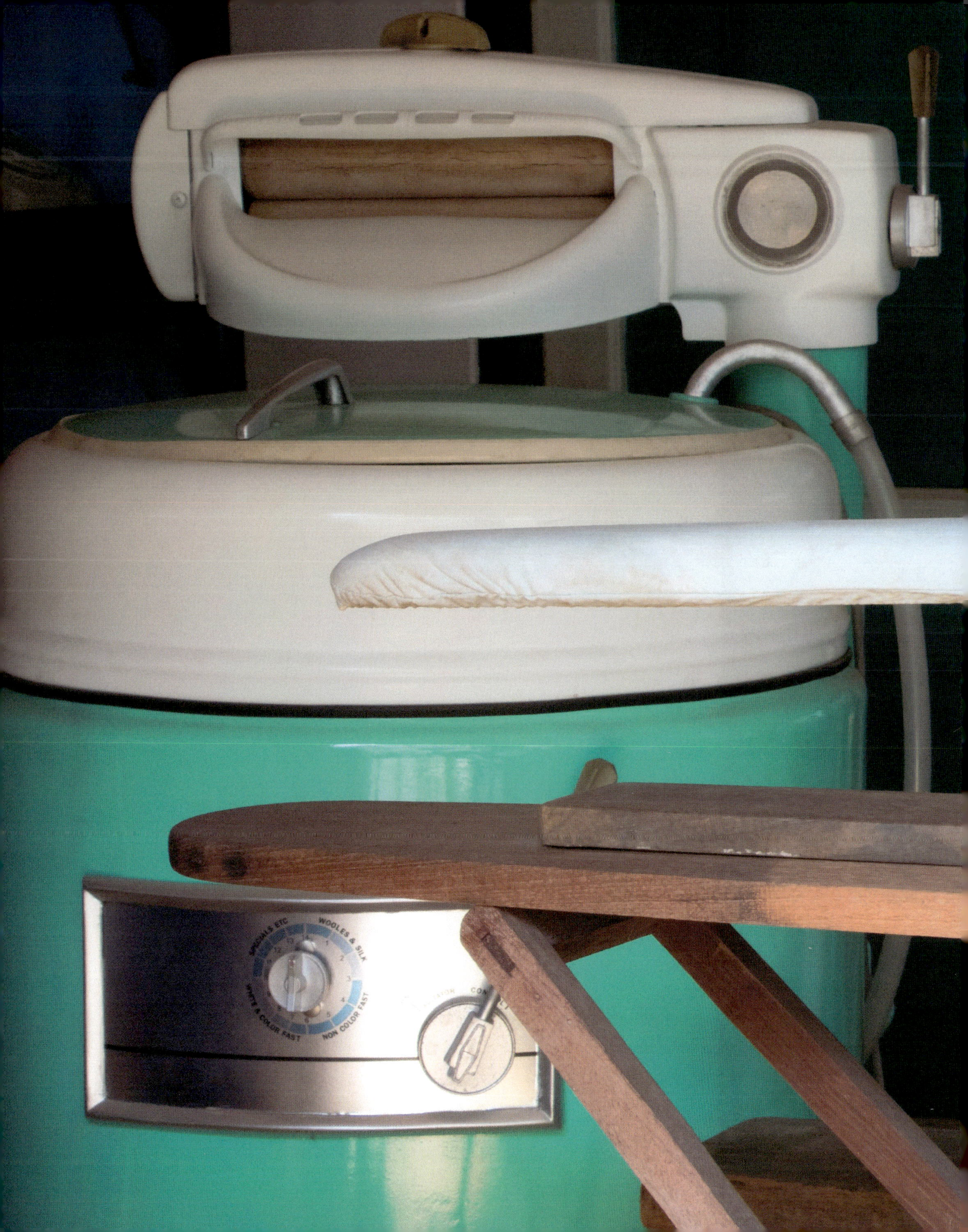
SPECIALS ETC
WOOLES & SILK
NON COLOR FAST
WHITE & COLOR FAST

Drying day

These days, if it's raining, you can pop a load of washing into the tumble dryer. We didn't have that option.

If it was sunny, the clothes were pegged outside on a line, or a rotary clothes hoist. Wooden clothes pegs, of course!

In gloomy weather, you might have a wooden clothes horse in front of the fire, or a drying rack that pulled up to the kitchen ceiling. Other people had electric airers, or airing cupboards. We all managed without electric dryers!

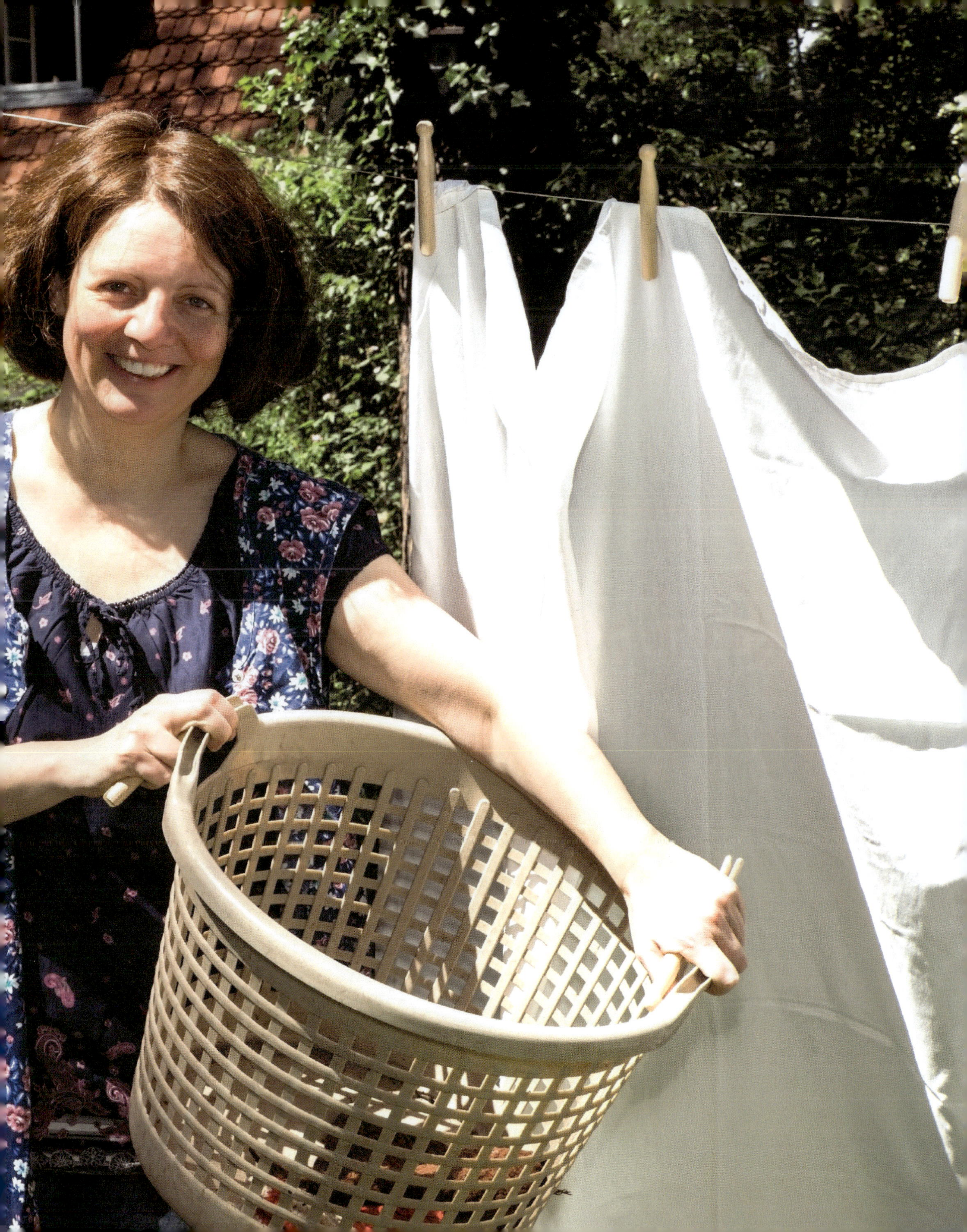

Ironing time

You might have had an ironing board, or just used an old table covered in a blanket and a cloth.

Everything got ironed, of course. Shirts, hankies, sheets, tablecloths – even cotton underwear!

In our house, we sometimes used spray starch, and a spray bottle of water was essential. We had a plain electric iron, so you had to dampen everything and use a pressing cloth. But at least we didn't have to use the old flat irons!

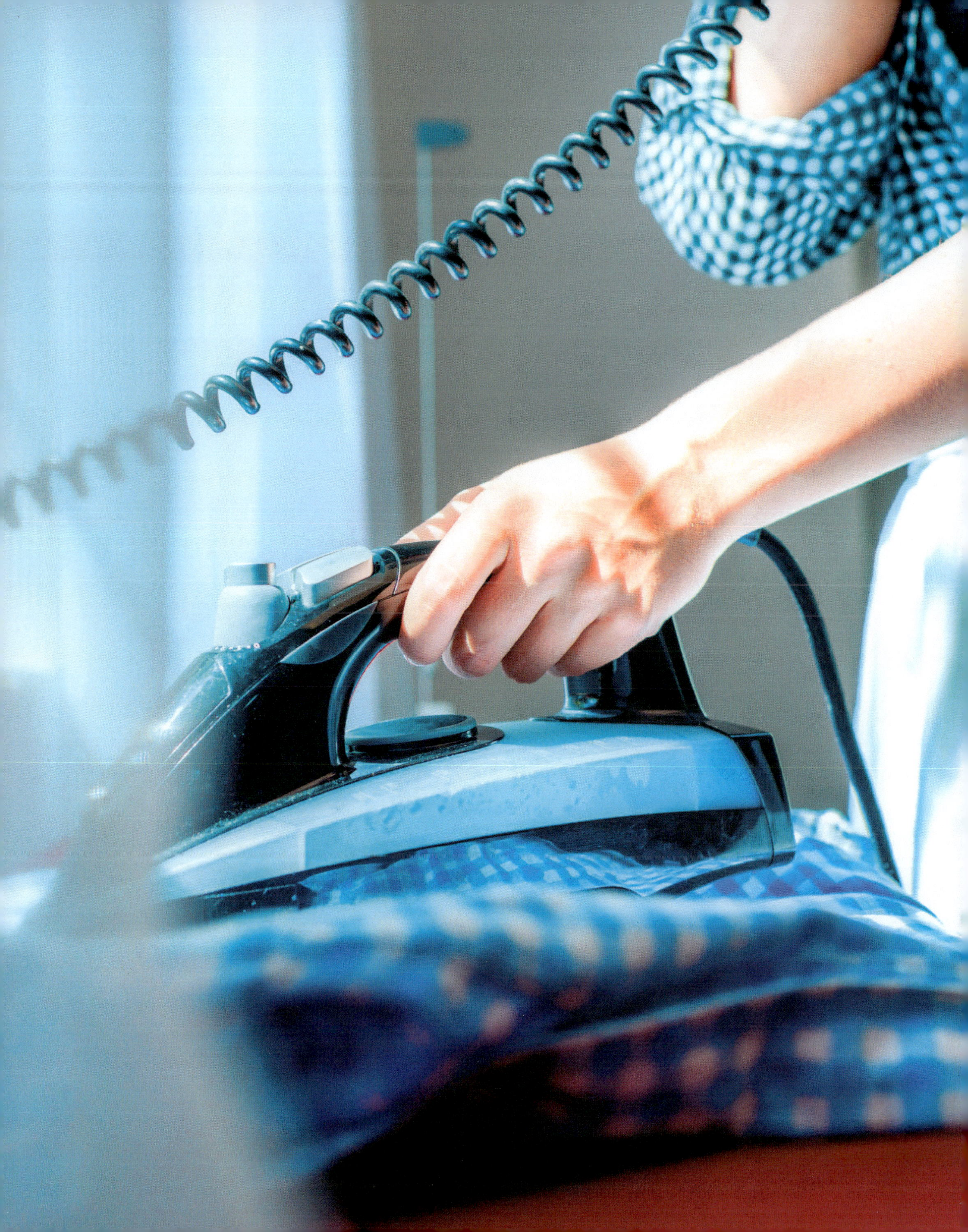

Cleaning routines

Magazines loved to tell housewives how to have a cleaning routine. I'm not sure everyone followed this, but many mothers did wash on Mondays.

Spring cleaning was a big thing, with all the furniture moved, ceilings and walls cleaned, curtains washed and rugs beaten.

Bedding could be left in the sunshine to air, while you cleaned the bed frame. I know many people still spring-clean, but we took it seriously back then!

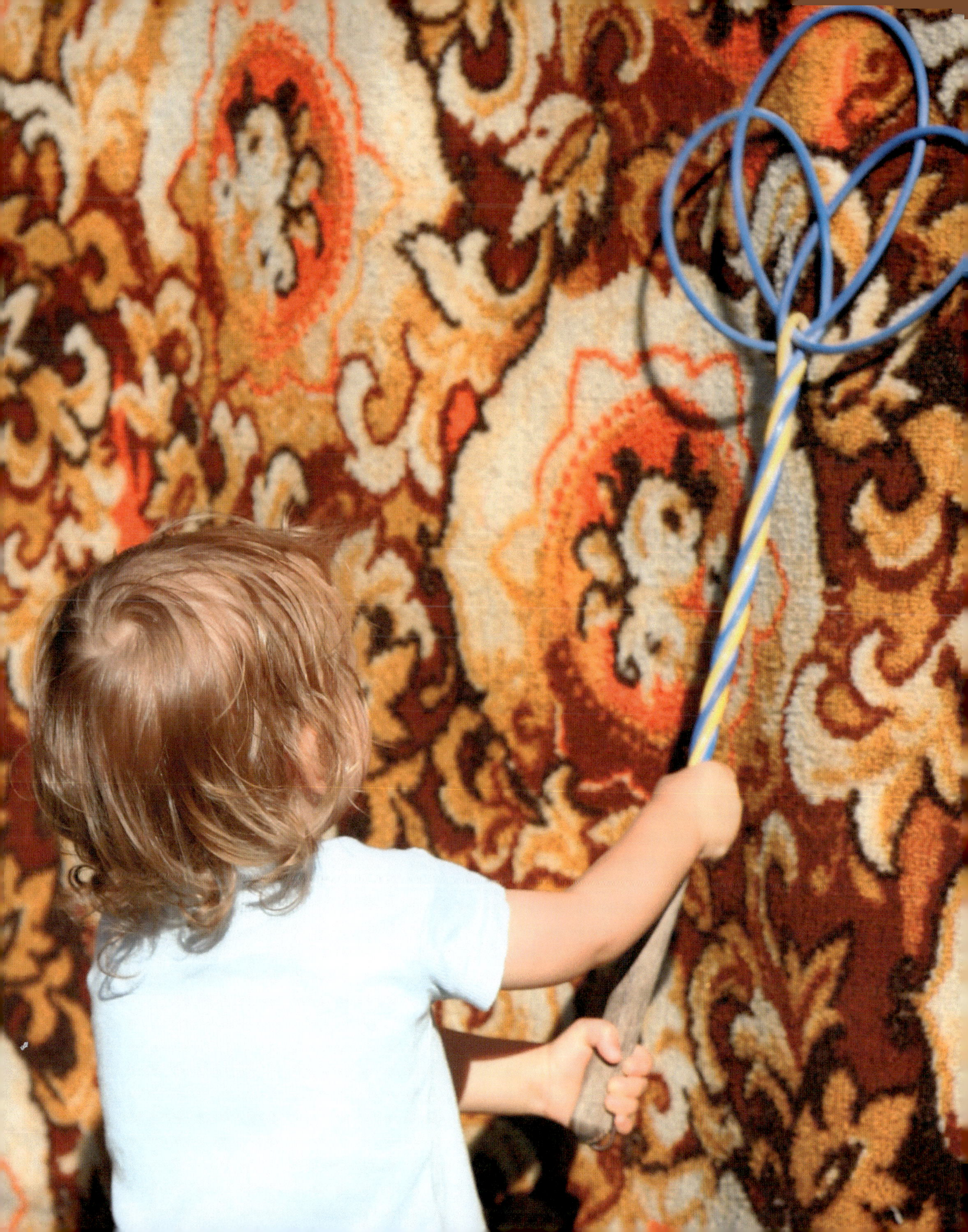

In the kitchen

Did you have a gas stove, electric – or an old wood range that kept the whole house warm?

Our house had gas, so we missed out on the experience of cleaning an old range, polishing the top and sweeping out ashes!

However, our stove-top did have to be dismantled for regular cleaning. That's when a little steel brush came in handy, plus scouring powder and steel wool.

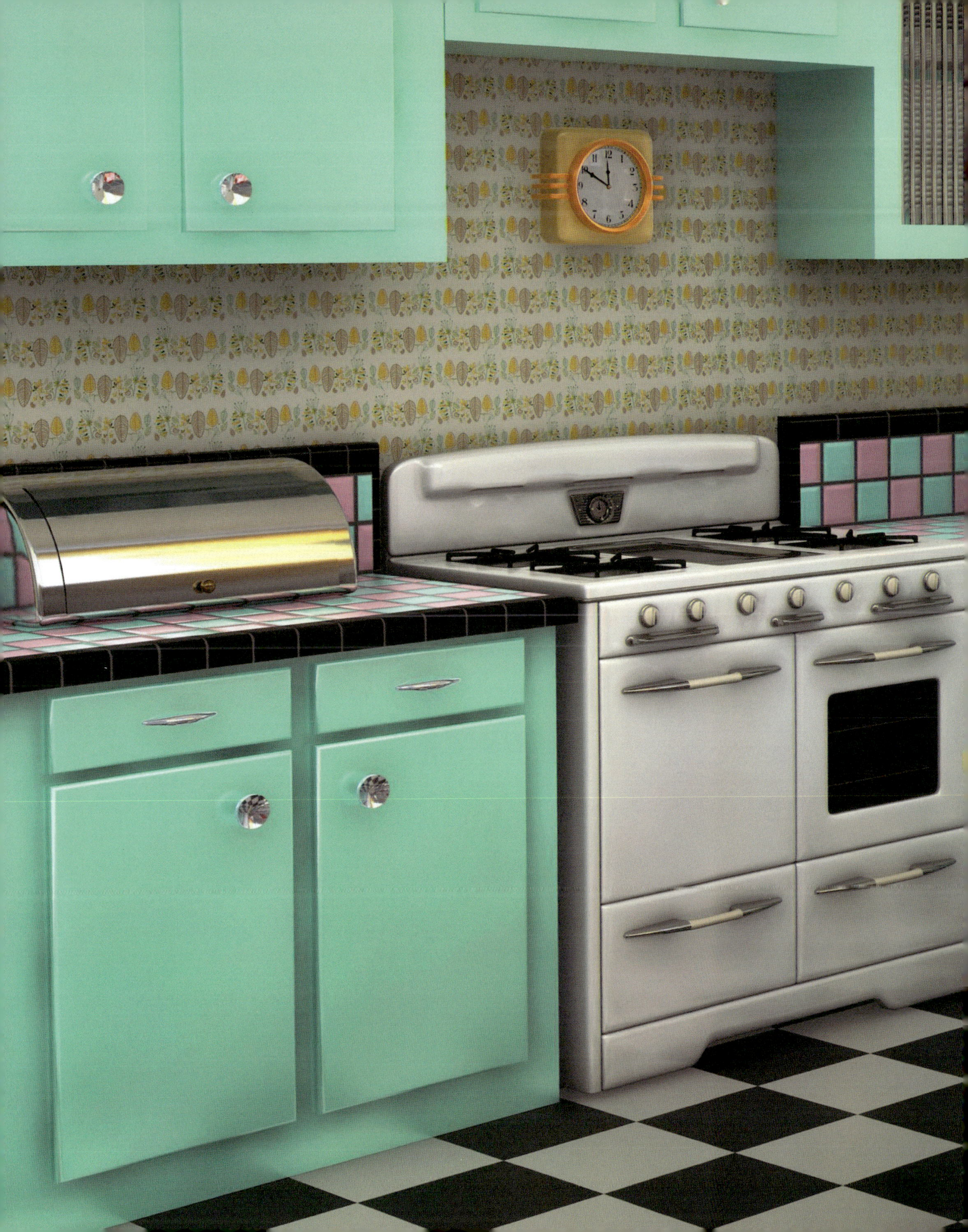

Keeping clean

Most people only had one bathroom, but then we didn't bath or shower as often as we do now. Some people still had an outside bathroom – or even a tin tub in the kitchen!

As kids, we often used strong-smelling soaps, like carbolic or coal tar, unless we'd been given bubble bath at Christmas. Soap on a rope came later!

Hair washing was a bit of a trial, with no conditioner. For girls, combing out long hair could be painful. Too many knots!

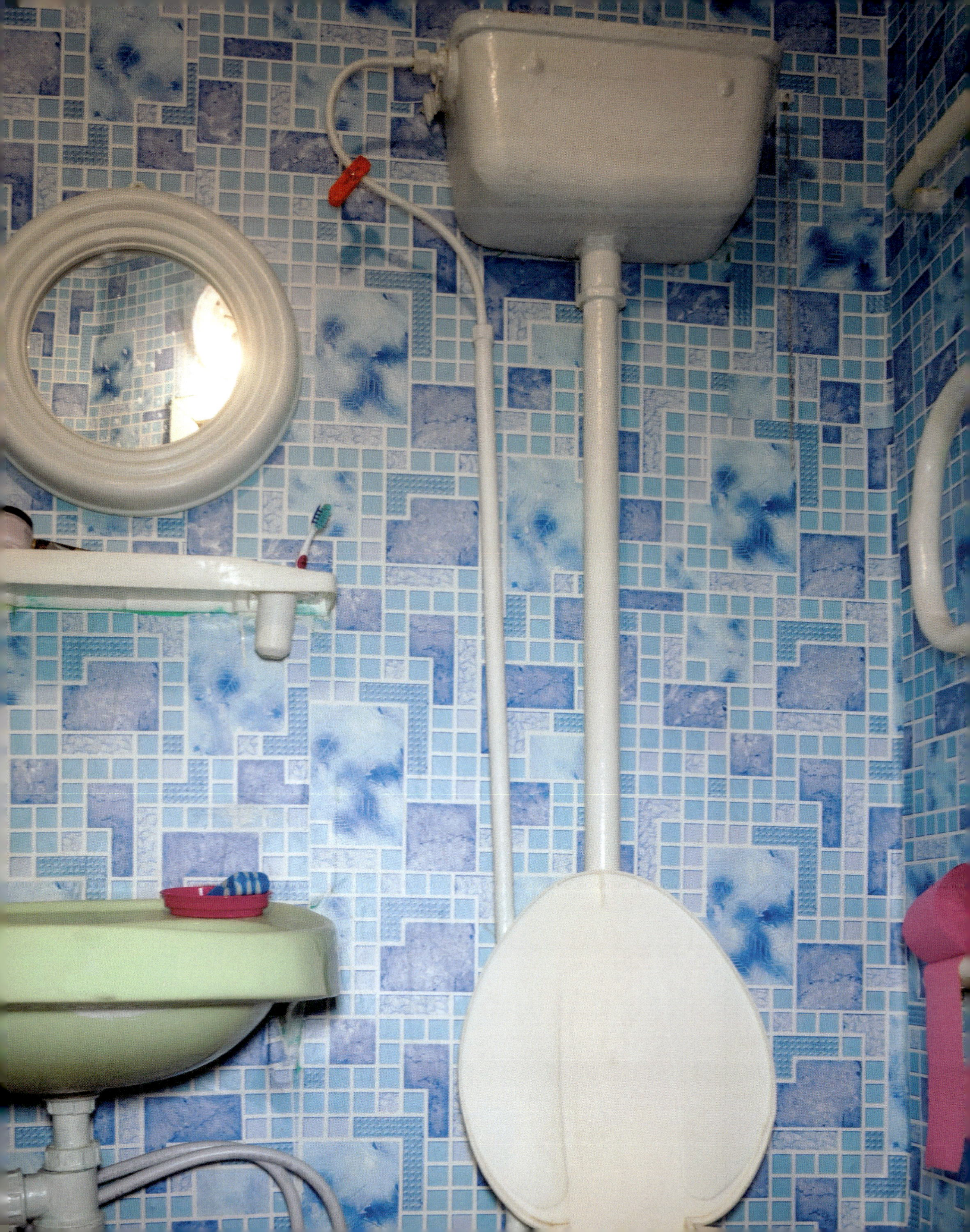

Washing dishes

Who washed the dishes in your home? Did you fight over whose turn it was to wash, whose turn to dry and put away?

I preferred drying. Those stiff linen tea-towels were boiled to keep them clean, so they soon became soft and supple.

For washing, we wore rubber gloves and used metal scourers to get the pots clean. Soap in a metal soap-saver eventually gave way to green dish-washing liquid. I know there were dishwashers, but I'd never seen one!

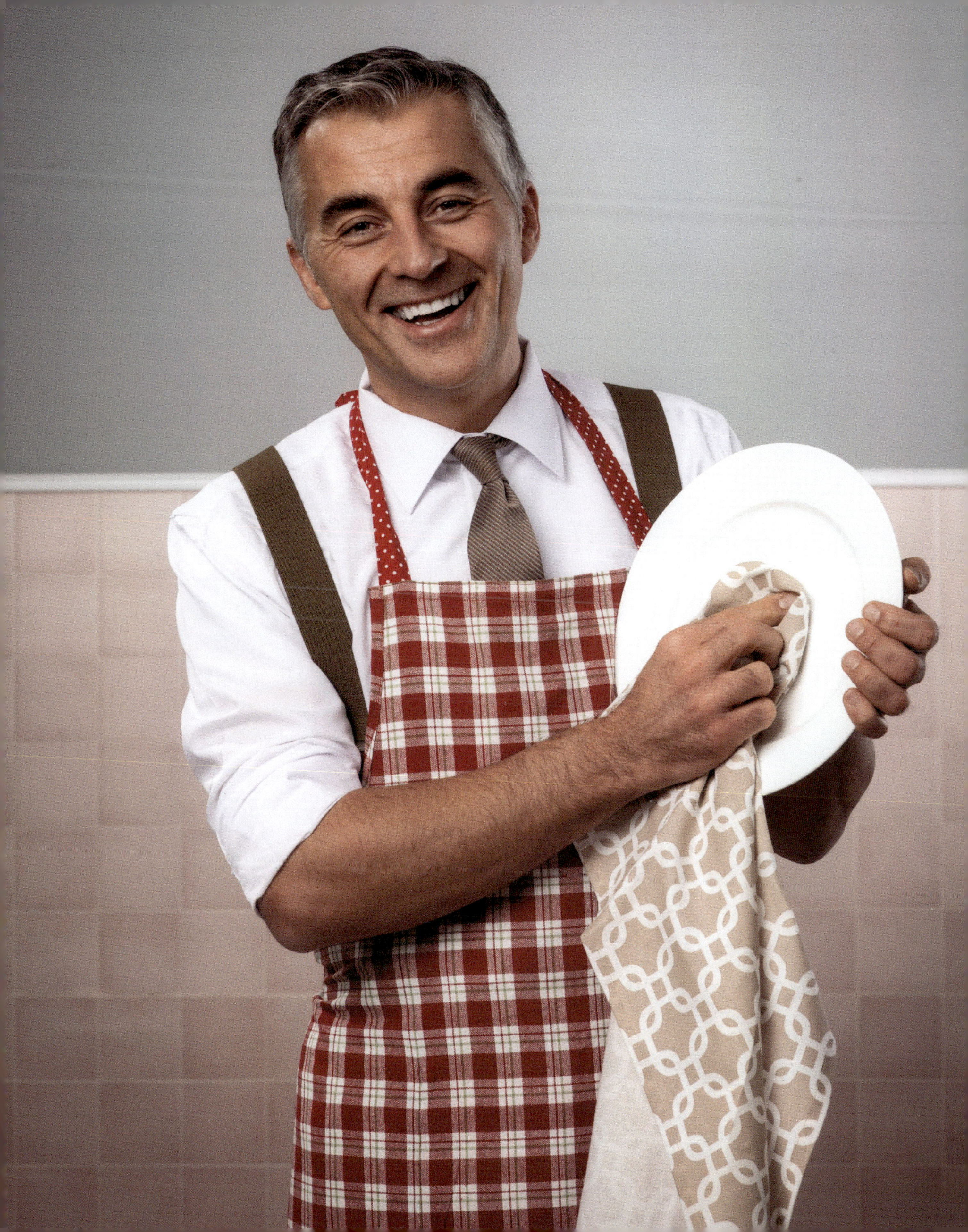

Dad jobs

There was more of a sense of 'women's work' and 'men's work' back then. Most men who were the 'breadwinners' didn't expect to be doing too much housework.

Men might do the washing up, plus household duties like cleaning shoes, winding the clock, or carving the roast.

Outside, it was a different story, with all manner of weekend jobs for the 'man of the house', including cleaning drains or gutters, washing the car if you had one, or mowing the lawn.

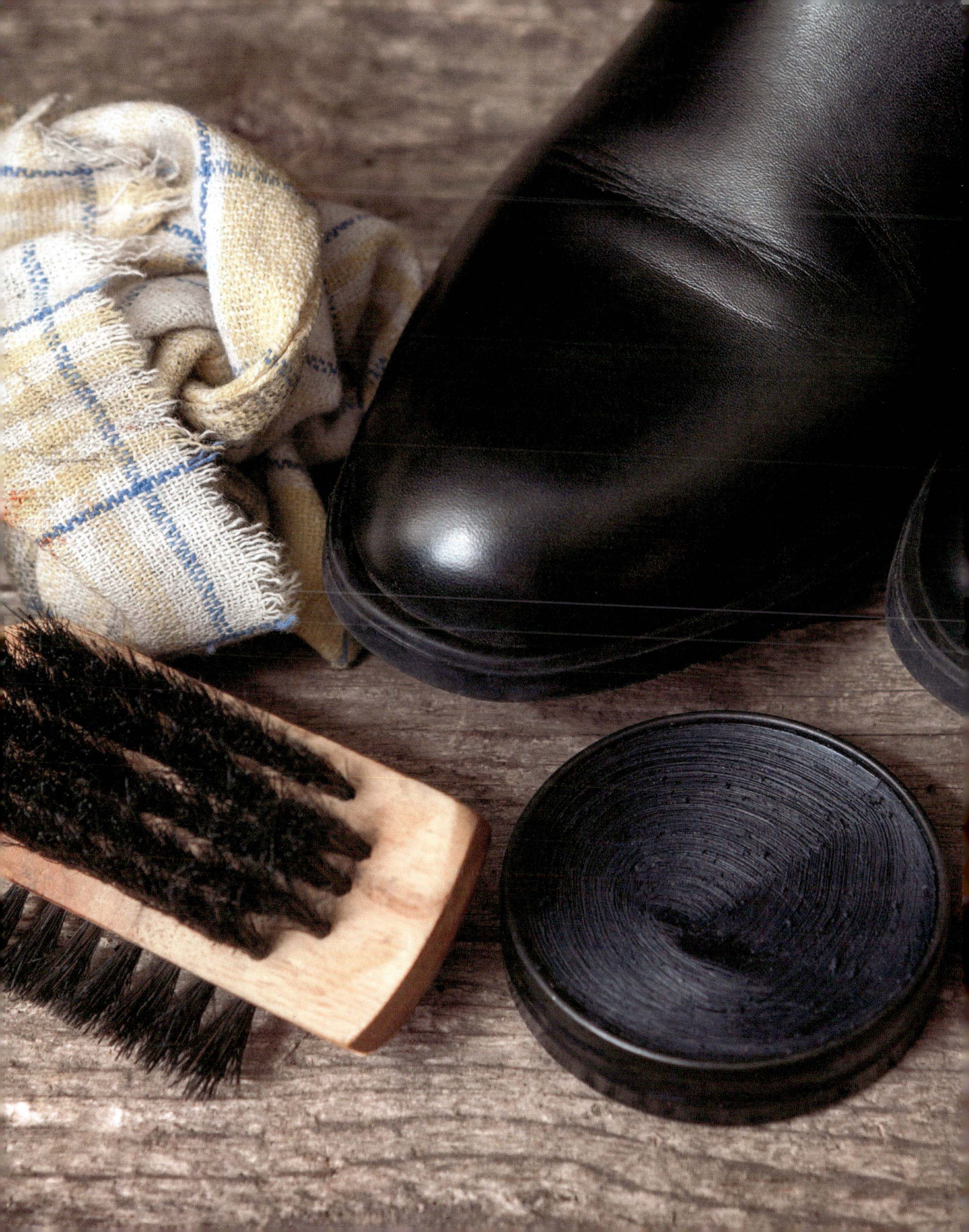

Rubbish

Without plastic bags, how did we keep the rubbish bin (or trash can) clean?

First of all, we didn't have so much to throw away, because there was far less packaging back then. Food scraps might feed chickens or pets, or be buried in the back yard as compost. Paper could go on the fire.

You lined your rubbish bin with old newspaper, and wrapped any wet scraps in more newspaper. The bin still needed a good regular clean, mind you!

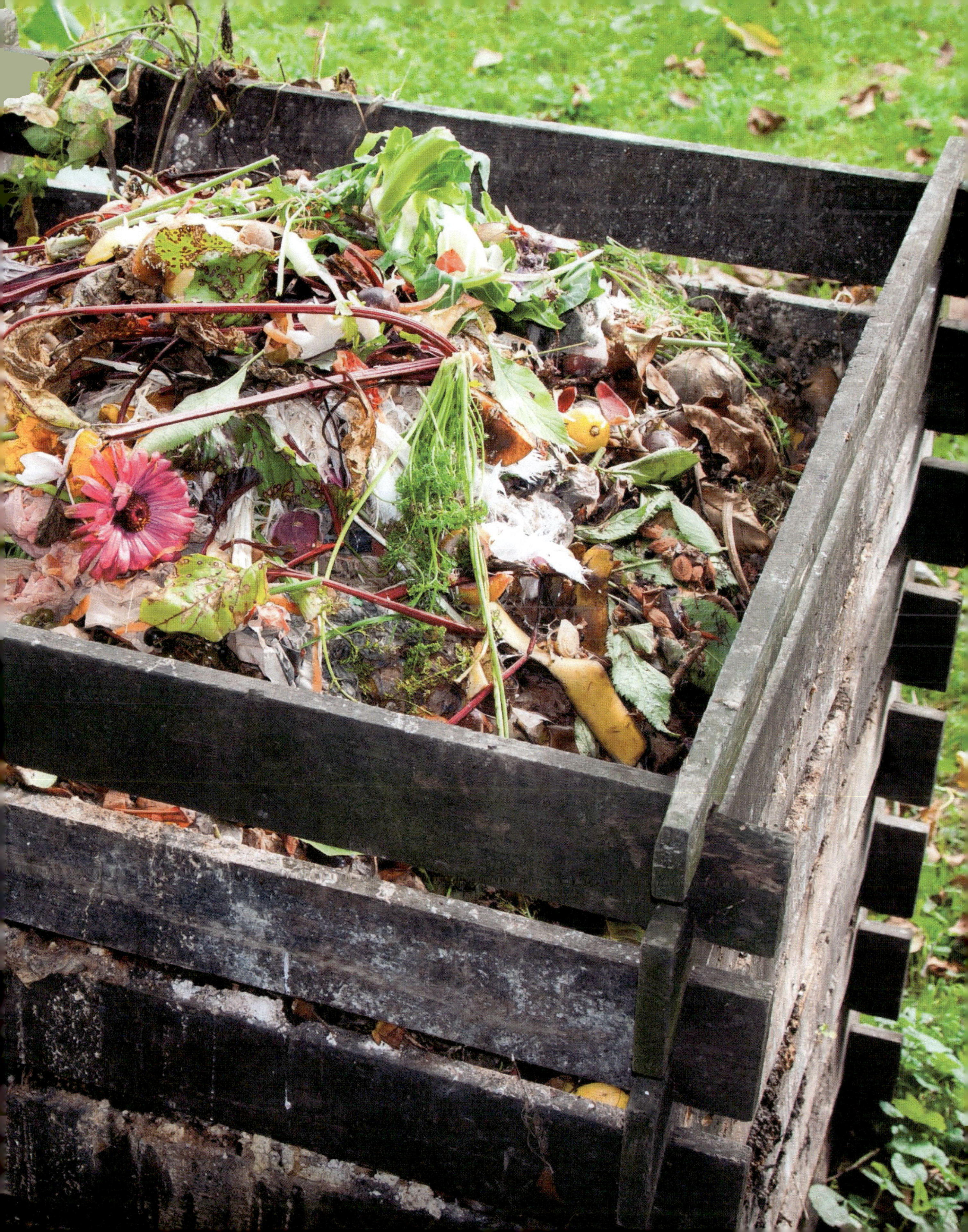

Household help

When my sister was born, we had a home help who came once a week to do the laundry. That would have been a real luxury for my mother.

Some people used a laundry service, or took their washing to a laundrette.

Not many ordinary people had a regular cleaner, though. That was the housewife's work, like it or not! Of course the family had to pitch in and help. There was plenty to do!

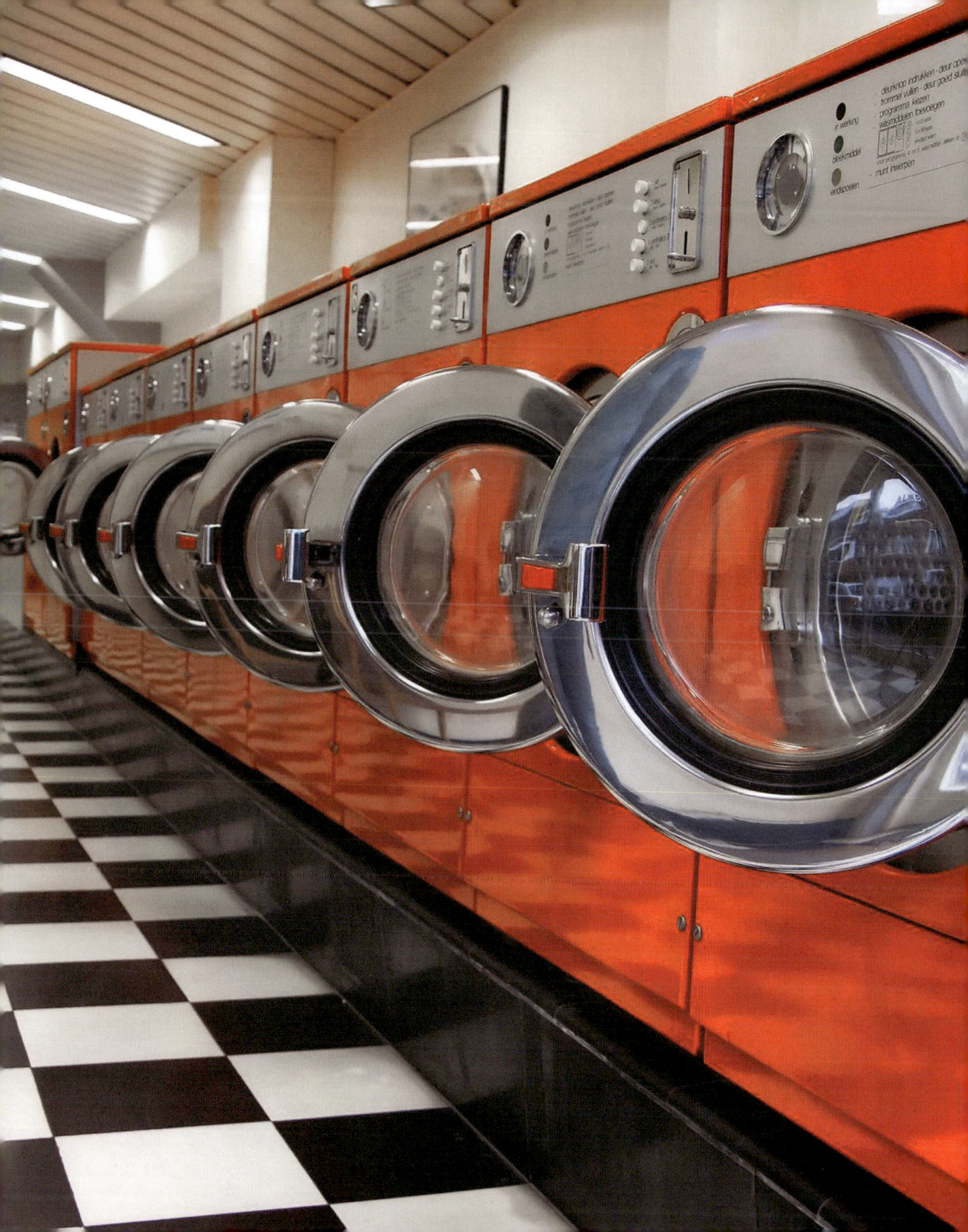
in werking
bleekmiddel
endspoelen
programma kiezen
wasmiddelen toevoegen
munt inwerpen

Mousetraps and mothballs

If you lived in an old house, you might be sharing it with unwanted wildlife. Birds falling down the chimney, perhaps? Australian friends had possums in the ceiling.

Everyone tried to keep their kitchen spotless, to keep mice away, but most people still put out mouse traps, even if they had a cat.

Clothes moths were another big problem. The answer – mothballs! That mothball smell took ages to air out, if it ever did!

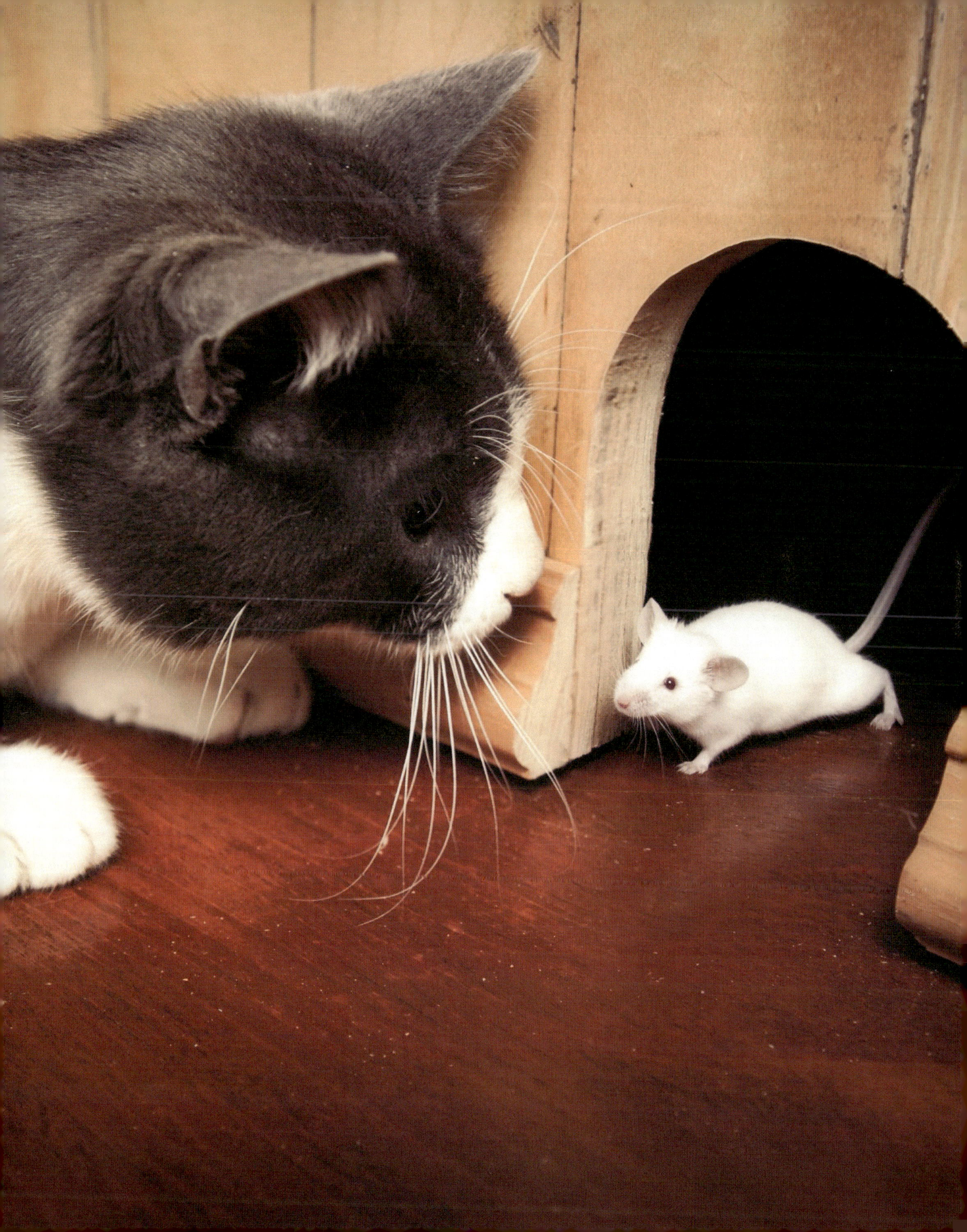

Keeping things nice

Visiting older people, you might see lace antimacassars on their sofas and armchairs, as protection from men's hair cream.

Everyone wanted to keep things nice. We covered up 'good stuff', and always wore a 'pinnie' while doing housework.

Of course, aprons weren't just to keep you clean. They were also a fashion statement, and could be the first thing you made in sewing class at school!

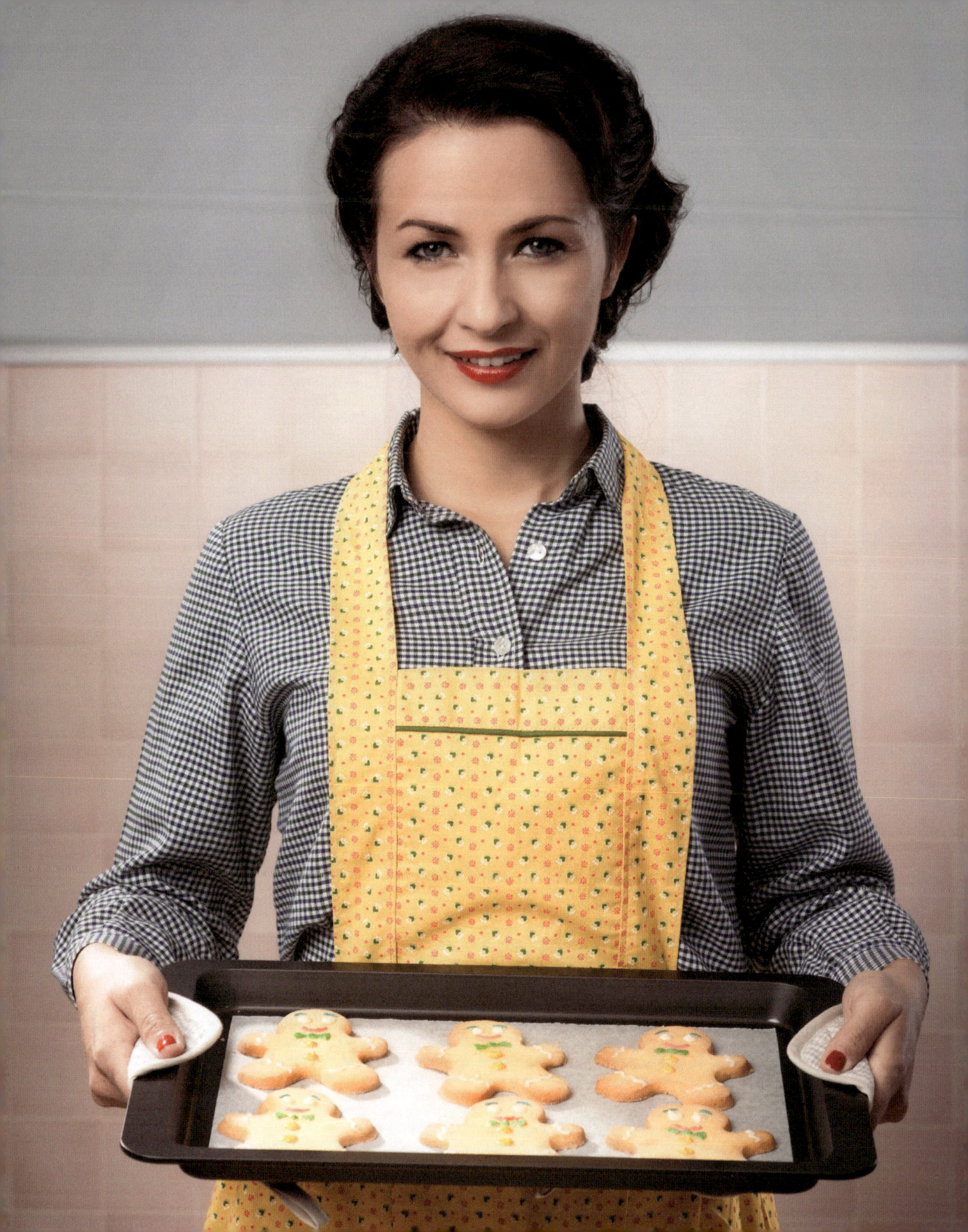

Household chores

As city kids, we had to help with the housework, wash dishes and keep our rooms clean.

Dusting was fun, but you might not be allowed to touch any treasures, in case you broke them. A less exciting job was cleaning out a budgie's cage.

Talk to a country kid however, and the story will be quite different. Carting water? Cleaning the hen-house, or all the work boots? That's probably true today as much as then!

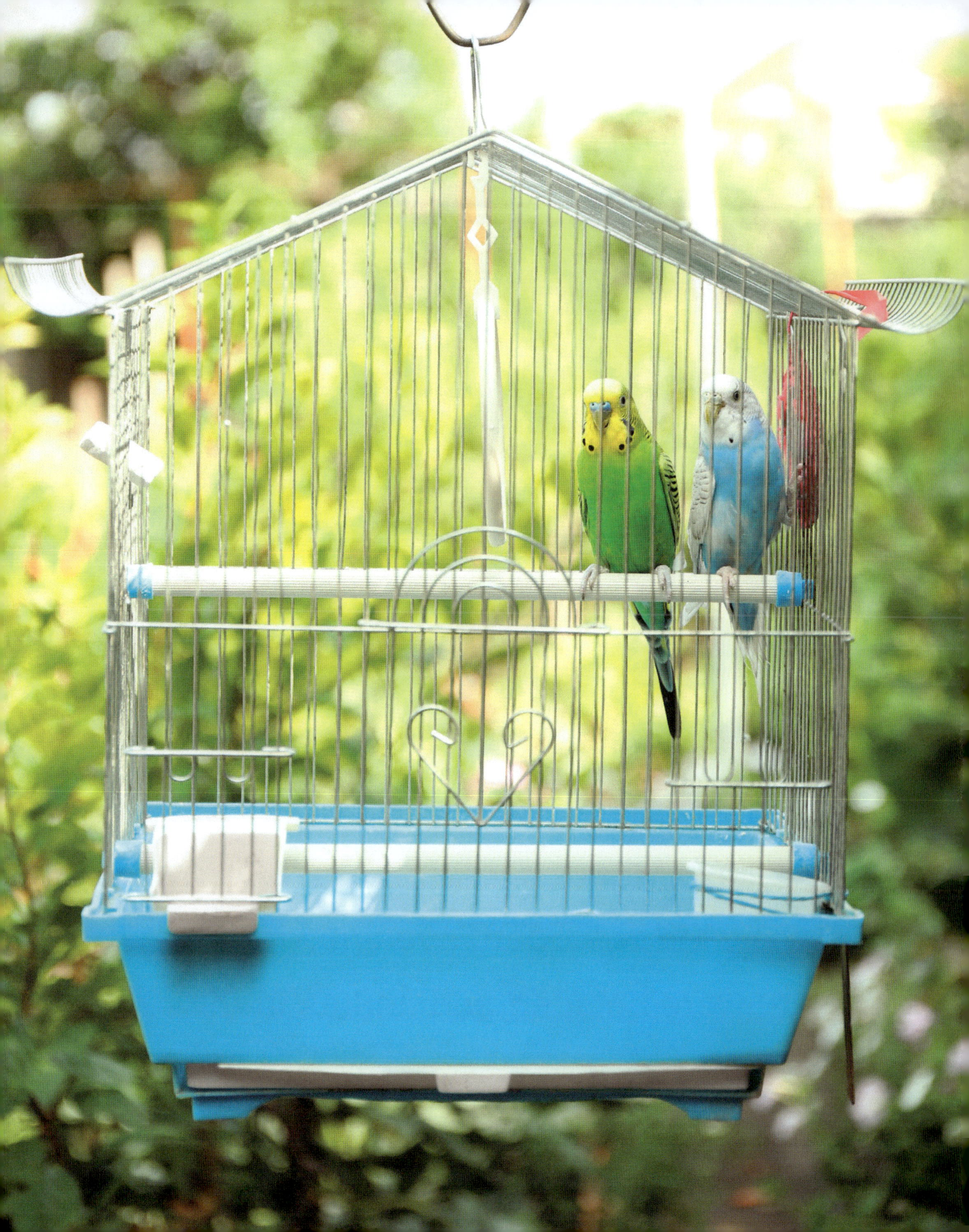

Ashtrays, ashtrays everywhere!

What can you see on the table? Yes, an ashtray! Ashtrays were everywhere, even in the car. Children made pottery ashtrays to give as gifts.

Even if you didn’t smoke, you had a few ashtrays in the house. At least they were easy to clean, but the smell of smoke lingered.

After any visitors had gone, we’d throw all the windows open, even in winter! There were no scented candles in those days!

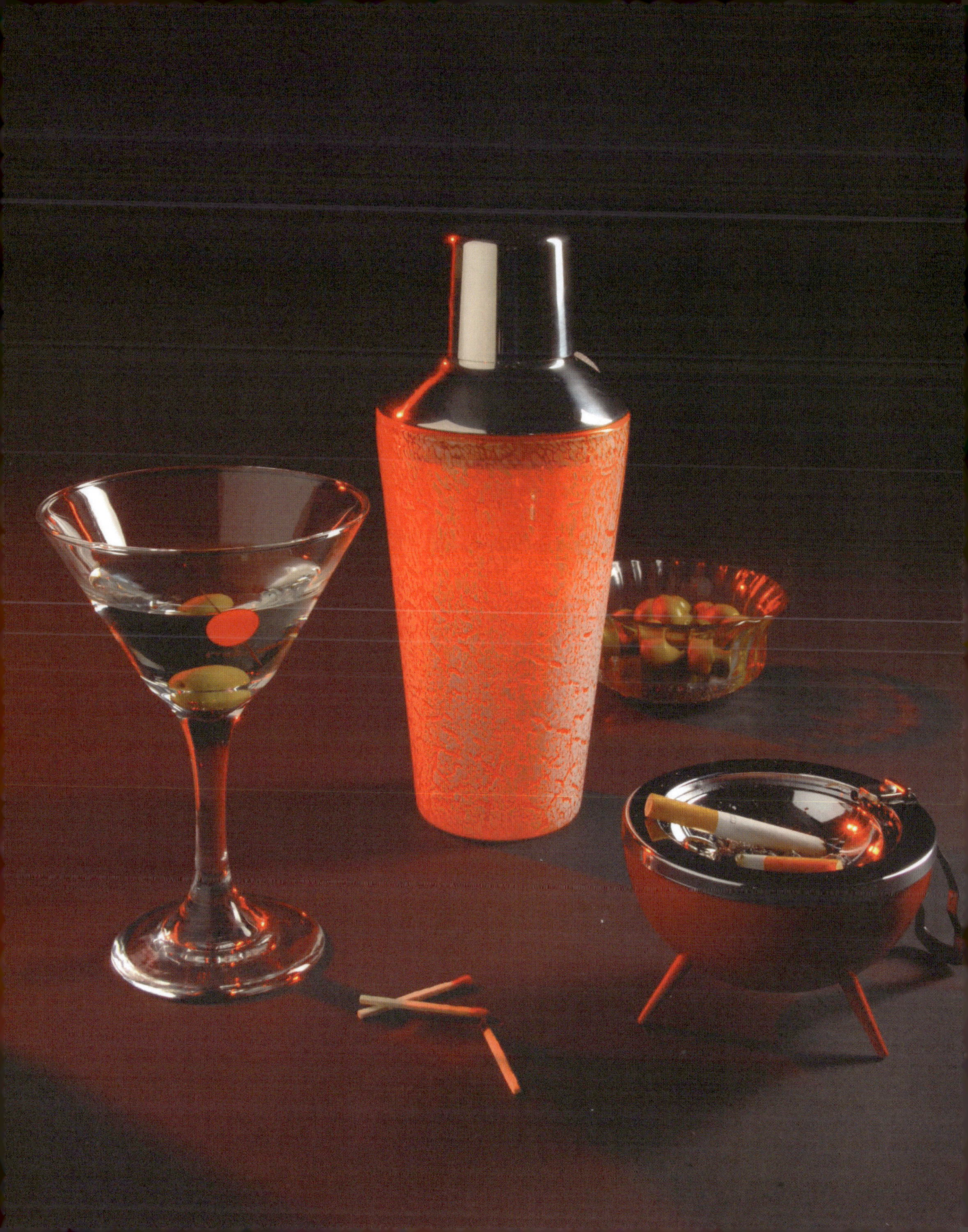

Looking back...

Reflecting on life back then, there are things I don't miss at all. So much scrubbing and polishing – and some chemicals we wouldn't use now!

That 'perfect housewife' role was very satisfying for some women – and very frustrating for others.

Taking pride in your home is important, though. Back then it didn't matter how big or small your home was, as long as you kept it nice, and that's still true.

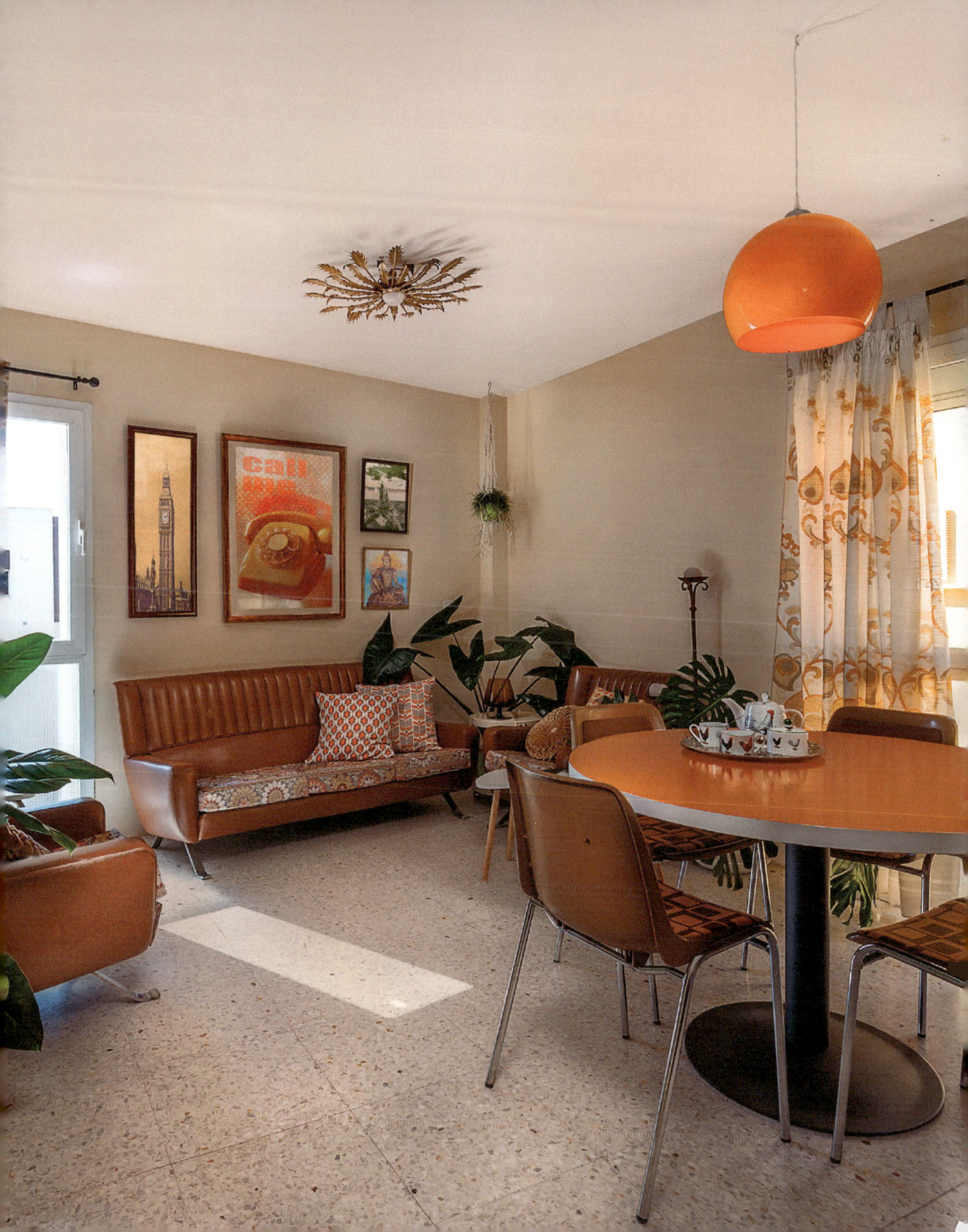
call
me

Thank you for reading and for sharing your own stories!

You might also enjoy:

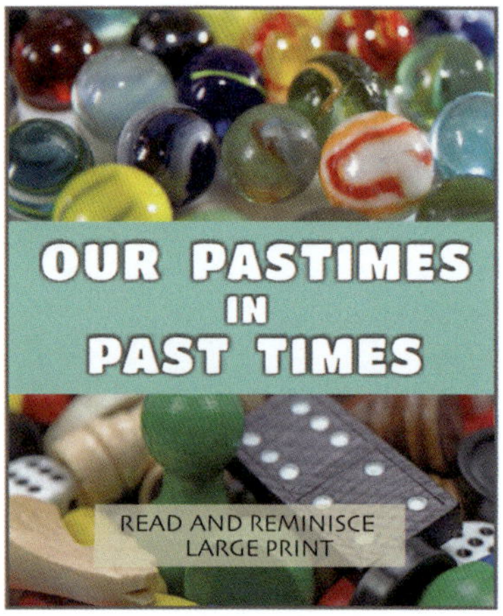

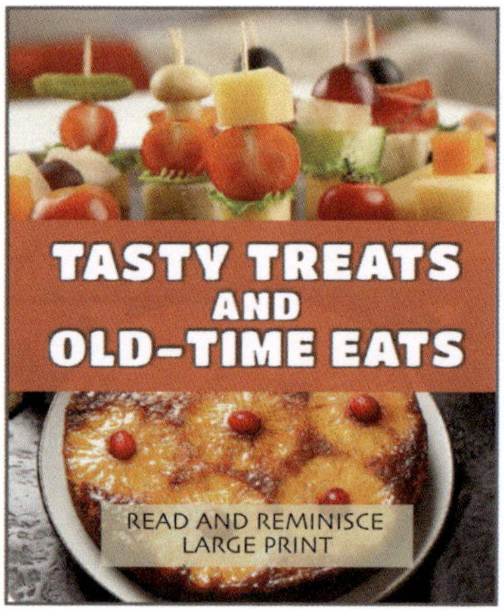

Huge thanks to Jennifer J. Barwick (series concept), Cora de la Cruz (professional advice), and to Elizabeth Bezant, Alison and Brendan Egan and all the wonderful editing team.

Photos thanks to Deposit Photos: Sandralise, londondeposit, ivonnewierink, PantherMediaSeller, Sandralise, norgallery, FotoHelin, wittayayut, Copit1606, AllaSerebrina, Hallgerd, jamesgroup, UncleDima, stokkete, cherriesjd, Airborne, PiXXart, fergregory, stokkete, belchonock, elroce and iStock Photos Valente Romero Sanchez

Printed in Dunstable, United Kingdom

66633035R00025